My Food Allergy Journal

If Lost, Return To:

_____

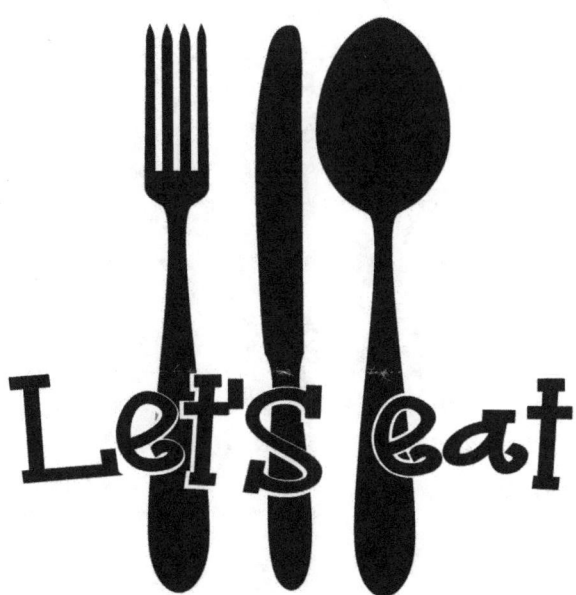

DEDICATION

This Food Allergy Diary Log is dedicated to all the people out there who want to record their food allergies and document their findings in the process.

You are my inspiration for producing books and I'm honored to be a part of keeping all of your food allergy notes and records organized.

This journal notebook will help you record your details about your food allergies.

Thoughtfully put together with these sections to record: Date, Time, Breakfast, Lunch, Dinner, Snacks, Symptoms & Reactions, Water Intake, & Notes.

HOW TO USE THIS BOOK

The purpose of this book is to keep all of your Food Allergy notes all in one place. It will help keep you organized.

This Food Allergy Diary Journal will allow you to accurately document every detail about your Food Allergies. It's a great way to chart your course through keeping track of your allergies.

Here are examples of the prompts for you to fill in and write about your experience in this book:

1. **Date** - Write the date.
2. **Time Of Day** - Log the time.
3. **Breakfast** - Record what you had for breakfast.
4. **Lunch** - Write what you had for lunch.
5. **Dinner** - Log what you had for dinner.
6. **Snacks** - Record any snacks you had.
7. **Symptoms & Reactions** - Write what your reactions & symptoms were.
8. **Water Intake** - Log the amount of water you drank.
9. **Notes** - Record any important information to note down related to your allergies such as exercise & fitness, body weight, calories intake, weight loss, personal sleep patterns, etc.

Date:_____

Breakfast	Time:	Symptoms/Reactions

Lunch	Time:	Symptoms/Reactions

Dinner	Time:	Symptoms/Reactions

Water Intake:

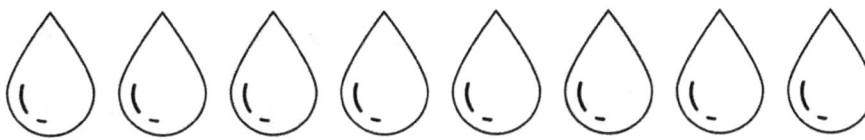

Snack 1 Time:	Symptoms/Reactions

Snack 1 Time:	Symptoms/Reactions

Snack 1 Time:	Symptoms/Reactions

Notes:

_____

_____

_____

_____

_____

Date:_____

Breakfast Time:	Symptoms/Reactions

Lunch Time:	Symptoms/Reactions

Dinner Time:	Symptoms/Reactions

Water Intake:

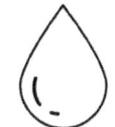 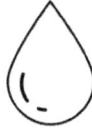 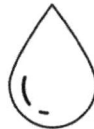 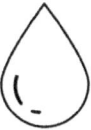 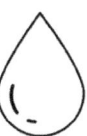 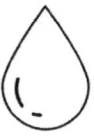 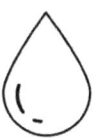 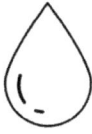

Snack 1 Time:	Symptoms/Reactions

Snack 1 Time:	Symptoms/Reactions

Snack 1 Time:	Symptoms/Reactions

Notes:

_____

_____

_____

_____

_____

Date:_____

Breakfast Time:	Symptoms/Reactions

Lunch Time:	Symptoms/Reactions

Dinner Time:	Symptoms/Reactions

Water Intake:

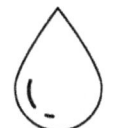 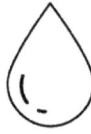 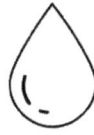 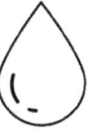 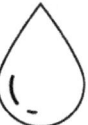 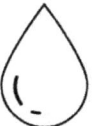 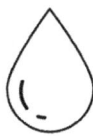 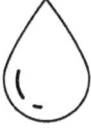

Snack 1 Time:	Symptoms/Reactions

Snack 1 Time:	Symptoms/Reactions

Snack 1 Time:	Symptoms/Reactions

Notes:

_____

_____

_____

_____

_____

Date:_____

Breakfast Time:	Symptoms/Reactions

Lunch Time:	Symptoms/Reactions

Dinner Time:	Symptoms/Reactions

Water Intake:

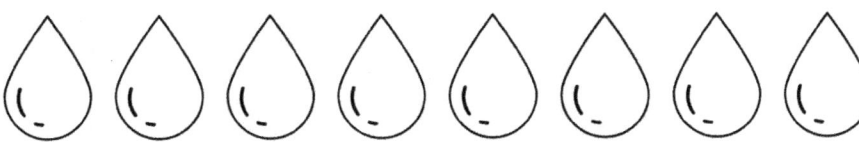

Snack 1 Time:	Symptoms/Reactions

Snack 1 Time:	Symptoms/Reactions

Snack 1 Time:	Symptoms/Reactions

Notes:

_____

_____

_____

_____

Date: _____

Breakfast Time:	Symptoms/Reactions

Lunch Time:	Symptoms/Reactions

Dinner Time:	Symptoms/Reactions

Water Intake:

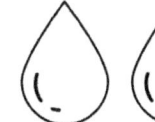 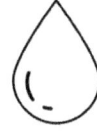 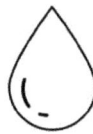 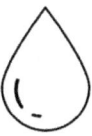 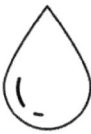 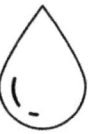 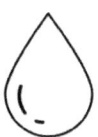 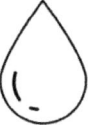

Snack 1 Time:	Symptoms/Reactions

Snack 1 Time:	Symptoms/Reactions

Snack 1 Time:	Symptoms/Reactions

Notes:

Date:_____

Breakfast Time:	Symptoms/Reactions

Lunch Time:	Symptoms/Reactions

Dinner Time:	Symptoms/Reactions

Water Intake:

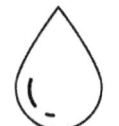 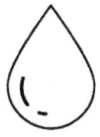 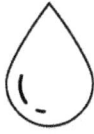 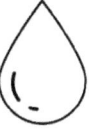 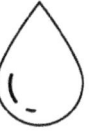 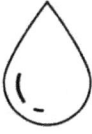 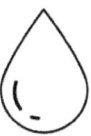 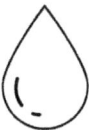

Snack 1 Time:	Symptoms/Reactions

Snack 1 Time:	Symptoms/Reactions

Snack 1 Time:	Symptoms/Reactions

Notes:

_____

_____

_____

_____

Date:_____

Breakfast Time:	Symptoms/Reactions

Lunch Time:	Symptoms/Reactions

Dinner Time:	Symptoms/Reactions

Water Intake:

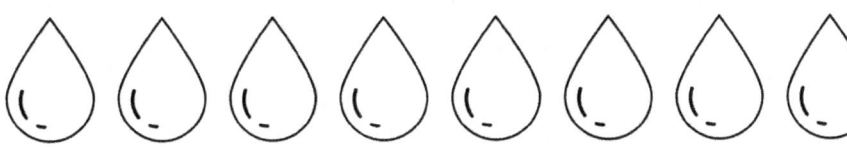

Snack 1 Time:	Symptoms/Reactions

Snack 1 Time:	Symptoms/Reactions

Snack 1 Time:	Symptoms/Reactions

Notes:

_____

_____

_____

_____

_____

Date:_____

Breakfast Time:	Symptoms/Reactions

Lunch Time:	Symptoms/Reactions

Dinner Time:	Symptoms/Reactions

Water Intake:

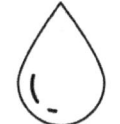 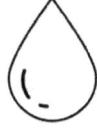 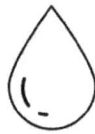 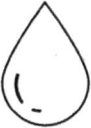 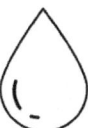 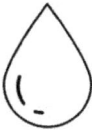 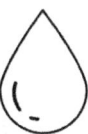 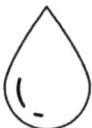

Snack 1 Time:	Symptoms/Reactions

Snack 1 Time:	Symptoms/Reactions

Snack 1 Time:	Symptoms/Reactions

Notes:

_____

_____

_____

_____

_____

Date:_____

Breakfast Time:	Symptoms/Reactions

Lunch Time:	Symptoms/Reactions

Dinner Time:	Symptoms/Reactions

Water Intake:

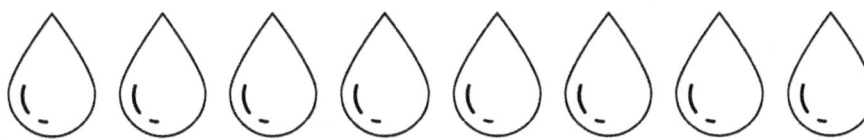

Snack 1 Time:	Symptoms/Reactions

Snack 1 Time:	Symptoms/Reactions

Snack 1 Time:	Symptoms/Reactions

Notes:

_____

_____

_____

_____

_____

Date:_____

Breakfast Time:	Symptoms/Reactions

Lunch Time:	Symptoms/Reactions

Dinner Time:	Symptoms/Reactions

Water Intake:

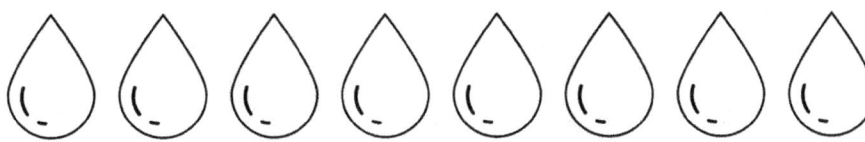

Snack 1 Time:	Symptoms/Reactions

Snack 1 Time:	Symptoms/Reactions

Snack 1 Time:	Symptoms/Reactions

Notes:

_____

_____

_____

_____

_____

Date:_____

Breakfast	Time:	Symptoms/Reactions

Lunch	Time:	Symptoms/Reactions

Dinner	Time:	Symptoms/Reactions

Water Intake:

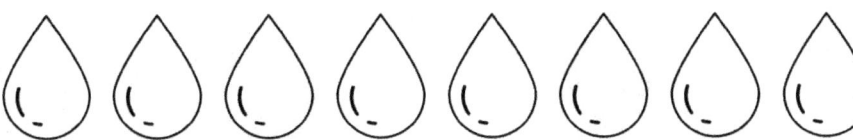

Snack 1 Time:	Symptoms/Reactions

Snack 1 Time:	Symptoms/Reactions

Snack 1 Time:	Symptoms/Reactions

Notes:

_____

_____

_____

_____

Date:_____

Breakfast Time:	Symptoms/Reactions

Lunch Time:	Symptoms/Reactions

Dinner Time:	Symptoms/Reactions

Water Intake:

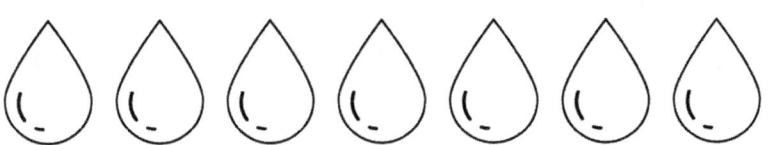

Snack 1 Time:	Symptoms/Reactions

Snack 1 Time:	Symptoms/Reactions

Snack 1 Time:	Symptoms/Reactions

Notes:

_____

_____

_____

_____

_____

Date:_____

Breakfast Time:	Symptoms/Reactions

Lunch Time:	Symptoms/Reactions

Dinner Time:	Symptoms/Reactions

Water Intake:

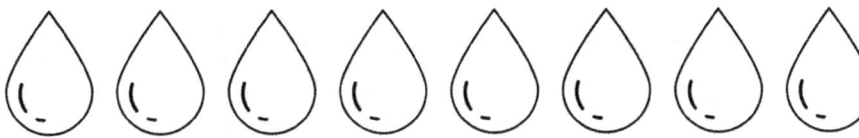

Snack 1 Time:	Symptoms/Reactions

Snack 1 Time:	Symptoms/Reactions

Snack 1 Time:	Symptoms/Reactions

Notes:

_____

_____

_____

_____

Date: _____

Breakfast Time:	Symptoms/Reactions

Lunch Time:	Symptoms/Reactions

Dinner Time:	Symptoms/Reactions

Water Intake:

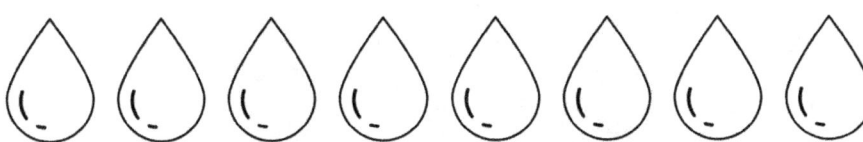

Snack 1 Time:	Symptoms/Reactions

Snack 1 Time:	Symptoms/Reactions

Snack 1 Time:	Symptoms/Reactions

Notes:

_____

_____

_____

_____

Date:_____

Breakfast Time:	Symptoms/Reactions

Lunch Time:	Symptoms/Reactions

Dinner Time:	Symptoms/Reactions

Water Intake:

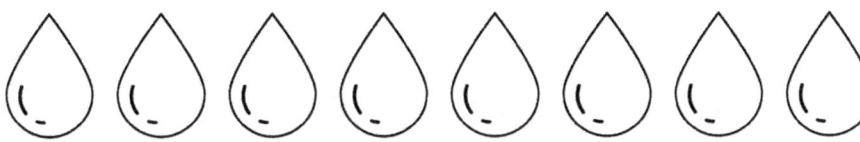

Snack 1 Time:	Symptoms/Reactions

Snack 1 Time:	Symptoms/Reactions

Snack 1 Time:	Symptoms/Reactions

Notes:

_____

_____

_____

_____

_____

Date:_____

Breakfast Time:	Symptoms/Reactions

Lunch Time:	Symptoms/Reactions

Dinner Time:	Symptoms/Reactions

Water Intake:

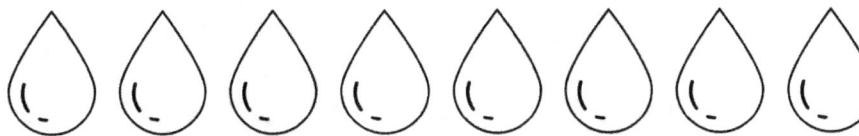

Snack 1 Time:	Symptoms/Reactions

Snack 1 Time:	Symptoms/Reactions

Snack 1 Time:	Symptoms/Reactions

Notes:

_____

_____

_____

_____

Date:_____

Breakfast Time:	Symptoms/Reactions

Lunch Time:	Symptoms/Reactions

Dinner Time:	Symptoms/Reactions

Water Intake:

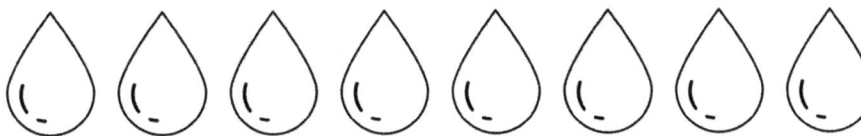

Snack 1 Time:	Symptoms/Reactions

Snack 1 Time:	Symptoms/Reactions

Snack 1 Time:	Symptoms/Reactions

Notes:

Date:_____

Breakfast Time:	Symptoms/Reactions

Lunch Time:	Symptoms/Reactions

Dinner Time:	Symptoms/Reactions

Water Intake:

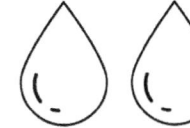 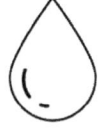 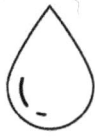 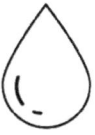  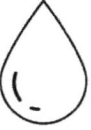 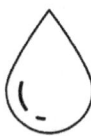 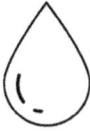

Snack 1 Time:	Symptoms/Reactions

Snack 1 Time:	Symptoms/Reactions

Snack 1 Time:	Symptoms/Reactions

Notes:

_____

_____

_____

_____

_____

Date:_____

Breakfast	Time:	Symptoms/Reactions

Lunch	Time:	Symptoms/Reactions

Dinner	Time:	Symptoms/Reactions

Water Intake:

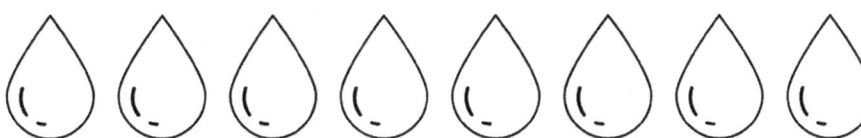

Snack 1 Time:	Symptoms/Reactions

Snack 1 Time:	Symptoms/Reactions

Snack 1 Time:	Symptoms/Reactions

Notes:

Date:_____

Breakfast Time:	Symptoms/Reactions

Lunch Time:	Symptoms/Reactions

Dinner Time:	Symptoms/Reactions

Water Intake:

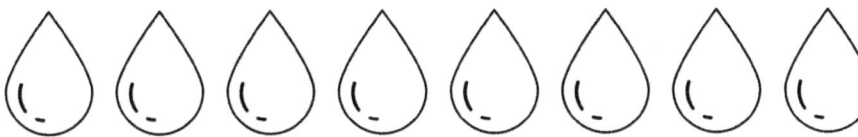

Snack 1 Time:	Symptoms/Reactions

Snack 1 Time:	Symptoms/Reactions

Snack 1 Time:	Symptoms/Reactions

Notes:

Date:_____

Breakfast Time:	Symptoms/Reactions

Lunch Time:	Symptoms/Reactions

Dinner Time:	Symptoms/Reactions

Water Intake:

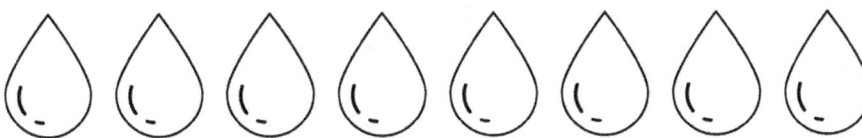

Snack 1 Time:	Symptoms/Reactions

Snack 1 Time:	Symptoms/Reactions

Snack 1 Time:	Symptoms/Reactions

Notes:

_____

_____

_____

_____

Date:_____

Breakfast Time:	Symptoms/Reactions

Lunch Time:	Symptoms/Reactions

Dinner Time:	Symptoms/Reactions

Water Intake:

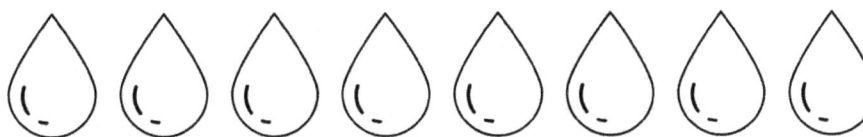

Snack 1 Time:	Symptoms/Reactions

Snack 1 Time:	Symptoms/Reactions

Snack 1 Time:	Symptoms/Reactions

Notes:

_____

_____

_____

_____

Date: _____

Breakfast Time:	Symptoms/Reactions

Lunch Time:	Symptoms/Reactions

Dinner Time:	Symptoms/Reactions

Water Intake:

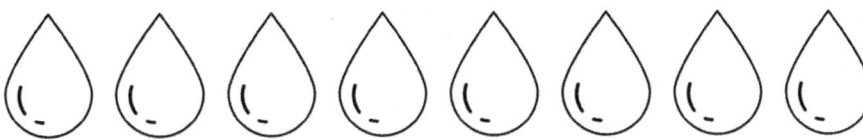

Snack 1 Time:	Symptoms/Reactions

Snack 1 Time:	Symptoms/Reactions

Snack 1 Time:	Symptoms/Reactions

Notes:

_____

_____

_____

_____

Date:_____

Breakfast Time:	Symptoms/Reactions

Lunch Time:	Symptoms/Reactions

Dinner Time:	Symptoms/Reactions

Water Intake:

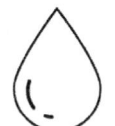 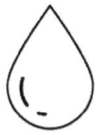 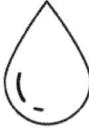 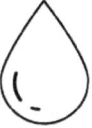 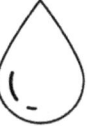 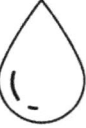 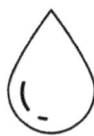 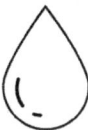

Snack 1 Time:	Symptoms/Reactions

Snack 1 Time:	Symptoms/Reactions

Snack 1 Time:	Symptoms/Reactions

Notes:

_____

_____

_____

_____

_____

Date:_____

Breakfast	Time:	Symptoms/Reactions

Lunch	Time:	Symptoms/Reactions

Dinner	Time:	Symptoms/Reactions

Water Intake:

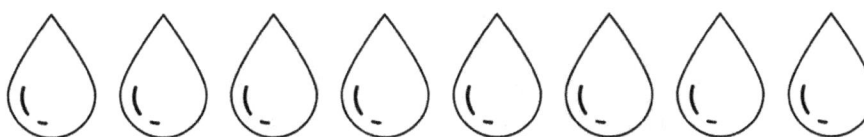

Snack 1 Time:	Symptoms/Reactions

Snack 1 Time:	Symptoms/Reactions

Snack 1 Time:	Symptoms/Reactions

Notes:

_____

_____

_____

_____

_____

Date:_____

Breakfast Time:	Symptoms/Reactions

Lunch Time:	Symptoms/Reactions

Dinner Time:	Symptoms/Reactions

Water Intake:

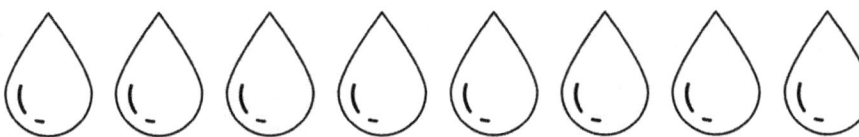

Snack 1 Time:	Symptoms/Reactions

Snack 1 Time:	Symptoms/Reactions

Snack 1 Time:	Symptoms/Reactions

Notes:

Date:_____

Breakfast Time:	Symptoms/Reactions

Lunch Time:	Symptoms/Reactions

Dinner Time:	Symptoms/Reactions

Water Intake:

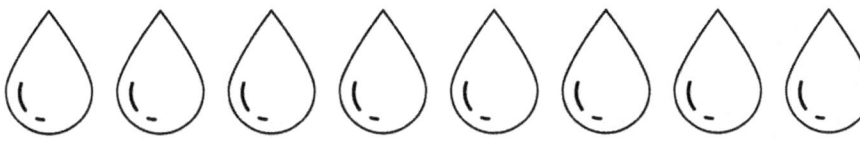

Snack 1 Time:	Symptoms/Reactions

Snack 1 Time:	Symptoms/Reactions

Snack 1 Time:	Symptoms/Reactions

Notes:

_____

_____

_____

_____

_____

Date:_____

Breakfast Time:	Symptoms/Reactions

Lunch Time:	Symptoms/Reactions

Dinner Time:	Symptoms/Reactions

Water Intake:

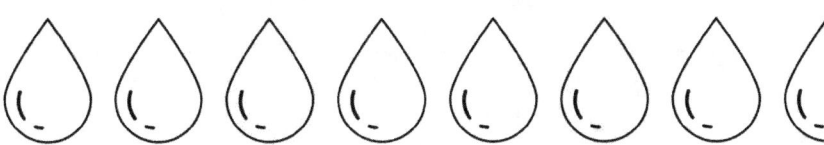

Snack 1 Time:	Symptoms/Reactions

Snack 1 Time:	Symptoms/Reactions

Snack 1 Time:	Symptoms/Reactions

Notes:

_____

_____

_____

_____

_____

Date:_____

Breakfast Time:	Symptoms/Reactions

Lunch Time:	Symptoms/Reactions

Dinner Time:	Symptoms/Reactions

Water Intake:

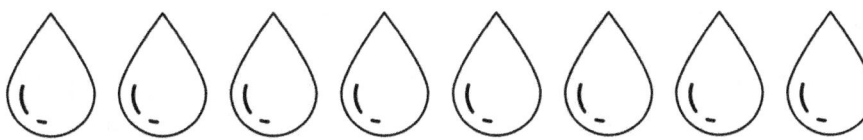

Snack 1 Time:	Symptoms/Reactions

Snack 1 Time:	Symptoms/Reactions

Snack 1 Time:	Symptoms/Reactions

Notes:

_____

_____

_____

_____

Date:_____

Breakfast Time:	Symptoms/Reactions

Lunch Time:	Symptoms/Reactions

Dinner Time:	Symptoms/Reactions

Water Intake:

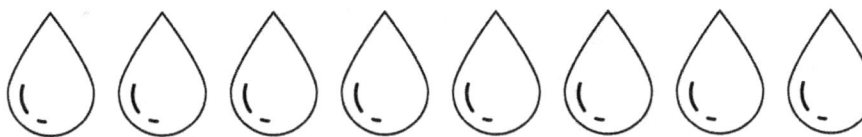

Snack 1 Time:	Symptoms/Reactions

Snack 1 Time:	Symptoms/Reactions

Snack 1 Time:	Symptoms/Reactions

Notes:

_____

_____

_____

_____

_____

Date:_____

Breakfast Time:	Symptoms/Reactions

Lunch Time:	Symptoms/Reactions

Dinner Time:	Symptoms/Reactions

Water Intake:

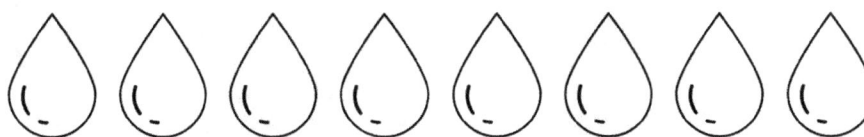

Snack 1	Time:	Symptoms/Reactions

Snack 1	Time:	Symptoms/Reactions

Snack 1	Time:	Symptoms/Reactions

Notes:

_____

_____

_____

_____

_____

Date:_____

Breakfast	Time:	Symptoms/Reactions

Lunch	Time:	Symptoms/Reactions

Dinner	Time:	Symptoms/Reactions

Water Intake:

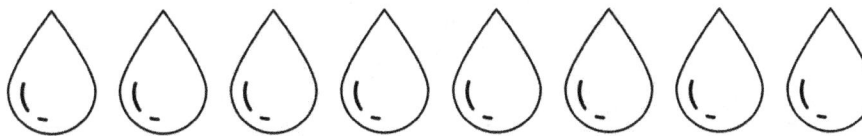

Snack 1 Time:	Symptoms/Reactions

Snack 1 Time:	Symptoms/Reactions

Snack 1 Time:	Symptoms/Reactions

Notes:

___
___
___
___

Date:_____

Breakfast Time:	Symptoms/Reactions

Lunch Time:	Symptoms/Reactions

Dinner Time:	Symptoms/Reactions

Water Intake:

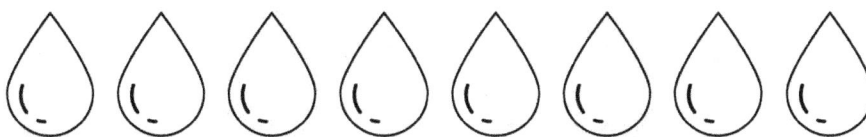

Snack 1 Time:	Symptoms/Reactions

Snack 1 Time:	Symptoms/Reactions

Snack 1 Time:	Symptoms/Reactions

Notes:

_____

_____

_____

_____

_____

Date:_____

Breakfast Time:	Symptoms/Reactions

Lunch Time:	Symptoms/Reactions

Dinner Time:	Symptoms/Reactions

Water Intake:

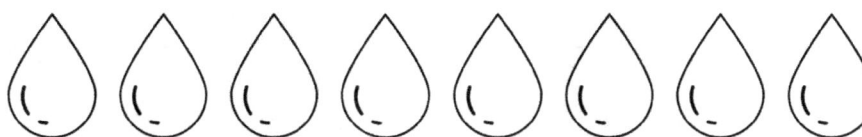

Snack 1 Time:	Symptoms/Reactions

Snack 1 Time:	Symptoms/Reactions

Snack 1 Time:	Symptoms/Reactions

Notes:

_____

_____

_____

_____

Date:_____

Breakfast Time:	Symptoms/Reactions

Lunch Time:	Symptoms/Reactions

Dinner Time:	Symptoms/Reactions

Water Intake:

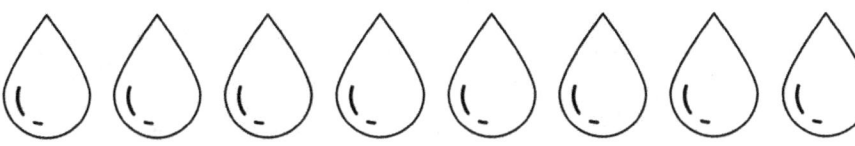

Snack 1 Time:	Symptoms/Reactions

Snack 1 Time:	Symptoms/Reactions

Snack 1 Time:	Symptoms/Reactions

Notes:

Date:_____

Breakfast　　Time:	Symptoms/Reactions

Lunch　　Time:	Symptoms/Reactions

Dinner　　Time:	Symptoms/Reactions

Water Intake:

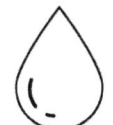 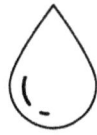 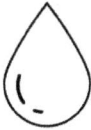 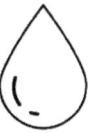 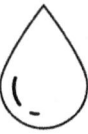 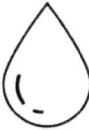 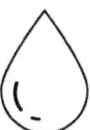 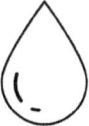

Snack 1 Time:	Symptoms/Reactions

Snack 1 Time:	Symptoms/Reactions

Snack 1 Time:	Symptoms/Reactions

Notes:

_____

_____

_____

_____

_____

Date:_____

Breakfast Time:	Symptoms/Reactions

Lunch Time:	Symptoms/Reactions

Dinner Time:	Symptoms/Reactions

Water Intake:

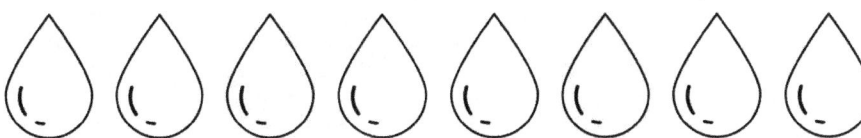

Snack 1 Time:	Symptoms/Reactions

Snack 1 Time:	Symptoms/Reactions

Snack 1 Time:	Symptoms/Reactions

Notes:

_____

_____

_____

_____

_____

Date:_____

Breakfast Time:	Symptoms/Reactions

Lunch Time:	Symptoms/Reactions

Dinner Time:	Symptoms/Reactions

Water Intake:

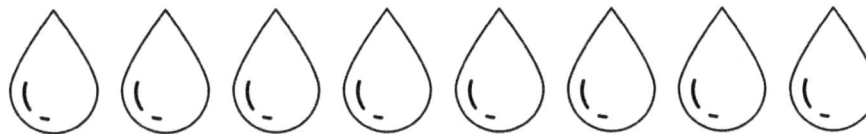

Snack 1 Time:	Symptoms/Reactions

Snack 1 Time:	Symptoms/Reactions

Snack 1 Time:	Symptoms/Reactions

Notes:

Date:_____

Breakfast	Time:	Symptoms/Reactions

Lunch	Time:	Symptoms/Reactions

Dinner	Time:	Symptoms/Reactions

Water Intake:

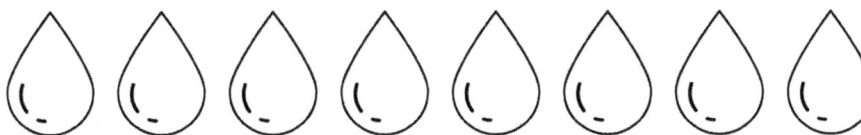

Snack 1 Time:	Symptoms/Reactions

Snack 1 Time:	Symptoms/Reactions

Snack 1 Time:	Symptoms/Reactions

Notes:

Date:_____

Breakfast	Time:	Symptoms/Reactions

Lunch	Time:	Symptoms/Reactions

Dinner	Time:	Symptoms/Reactions

Water Intake:

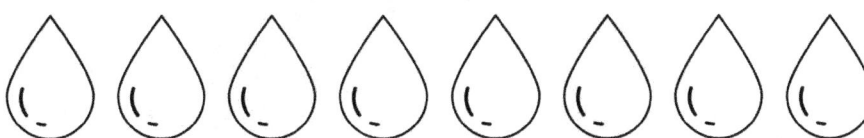

Snack 1 Time:	Symptoms/Reactions

Snack 1 Time:	Symptoms/Reactions

Snack 1 Time:	Symptoms/Reactions

Notes:

_____

_____

_____

_____

_____

Date: _____

Breakfast	Time:	Symptoms/Reactions

Lunch	Time:	Symptoms/Reactions

Dinner	Time:	Symptoms/Reactions

Water Intake:

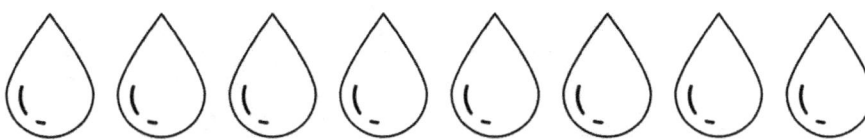

Snack 1 Time:	Symptoms/Reactions

Snack 1 Time:	Symptoms/Reactions

Snack 1 Time:	Symptoms/Reactions

Notes:

_____

_____

_____

_____

Date:_____

Breakfast Time:	Symptoms/Reactions

Lunch Time:	Symptoms/Reactions

Dinner Time:	Symptoms/Reactions

Water Intake:

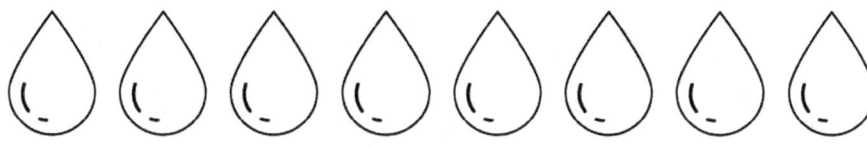

Snack 1 Time:	Symptoms/Reactions

Snack 1 Time:	Symptoms/Reactions

Snack 1 Time:	Symptoms/Reactions

Notes:

_____

_____

_____

_____

_____

Date:_____

Breakfast Time:	Symptoms/Reactions

Lunch Time:	Symptoms/Reactions

Dinner Time:	Symptoms/Reactions

Water Intake:

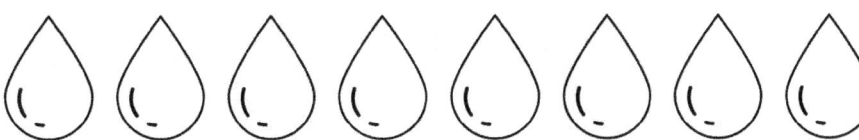

Snack 1 Time:	Symptoms/Reactions

Snack 1 Time:	Symptoms/Reactions

Snack 1 Time:	Symptoms/Reactions

Notes:

_____

_____

_____

_____

Date:_____

Breakfast	Time:	Symptoms/Reactions

Lunch	Time:	Symptoms/Reactions

Dinner	Time:	Symptoms/Reactions

Water Intake:

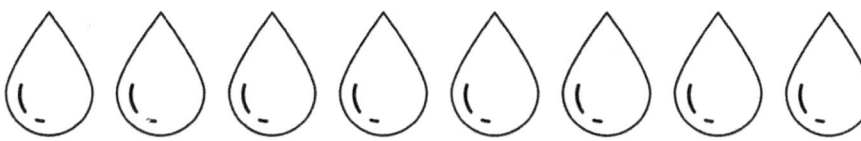

Snack 1 Time:	Symptoms/Reactions

Snack 1 Time:	Symptoms/Reactions

Snack 1 Time:	Symptoms/Reactions

Notes:

_____

_____

_____

_____

_____

Date:_____

Breakfast Time:	Symptoms/Reactions

Lunch Time:	Symptoms/Reactions

Dinner Time:	Symptoms/Reactions

Water Intake:

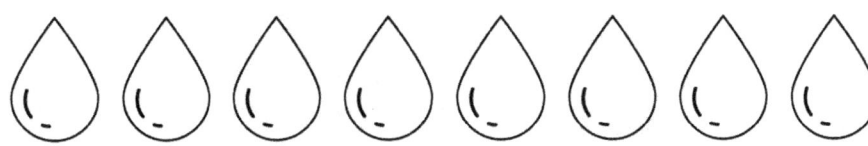

Snack 1 Time:	Symptoms/Reactions

Snack 1 Time:	Symptoms/Reactions

Snack 1 Time:	Symptoms/Reactions

Notes:

www.ingramcontent.com/pod-product-compliance
Lightning Source LLC
Chambersburg PA
CBHW071409080526
44587CB00017B/3232